AVIAN INFLUENZA:

A Comprehensive Guide for Health and Safety

LEONARD J. GREEN

DISCLAIMER

Copyright © by LEONARD J. GREEN 2024. All rights reserved.

Before this document is duplicated or reproduced in any manner, the publisher's consent must be gained.

Therefore, the contents within can neither be stored electronically, transferred, nor kept in a database. Neither in Part nor full can the document be copied, scanned, faxed, or retained without approval from the publisher or creator

TABLE OF CONTENT

Contents

DISCLAIMER 2
INTRODUCTION 4
A Brief Overview of Avian Influenza 4
Historical Background and Outbreaks 6
The Importance of Understanding Avian Influenza Today 7
CHAPTER 1 9
UNDERSTANDING AVIAN INFLUENZA VIRUS 9
Structure and Characteristics of the Avian Influenza Virus 9
Different strains and subtypes 11
Transmission and Spread of Avian Influenza 12
CHAPTER 2 14
SYMPTOMS AND CLINICAL MANIFESTATIONS 14
Signs and Symptoms in Avian Species 14
Human Infections: Symptoms and Complications 16
Variations in Clinical Presentation 18
CHAPTER 3 20
DIAGNOSIS AND DETECTION 20
Laboratory Tests for Avian Influenza 20
Diagnostic Methods in Humans and Animals 22
Challenges in Early Detection and Diagnosis 23
CHAPTER 4 26
PREVENTION AND CONTROL MEASURES 26

Vaccination Strategies for Poultry ... 26
Biosecurity Measures in Poultry Farms ... 28
Public Health Measures for Preventing Human Transmission ... 30
CHAPTER 5 ... 33
TREATMENT AND MANAGEMENT ... 33
Antiviral Medications for Avian Influenza ... 33
Supportive care for infected individuals ... 35
Strategies for Managing Outbreaks in Poultry and Humans ... 37
CHAPTER 6 ... 40
GLOBAL SURVEILLANCE AND RESPONSE ... 40
International Efforts in Monitoring Avian Influenza ... 41
Collaborative Response Mechanisms ... 42
Challenges and Opportunities in Global Surveillance ... 44
CHAPTER 7 ... 46
PUBLIC HEALTH PREPAREDNESS ... 46
National and Regional Preparedness Plans ... 46
Role of Healthcare Providers in Surveillance and Response ... 49
Community Education and Awareness Programs ... 50
CHAPTER 8 ... 53
ONE HEALTH APPROACH ... 53
Integrating human, animal, and environmental health ... 54
Importance of Collaboration and Interdisciplinary Efforts ... 55
Case Studies and Success Stories ... 57
CHAPTER 9 ... 60
FUTURE PERSPECTIVES AND EMERGING CHALLENGES
... 60

Evolutionary Trends in the Avian Influenza Virus 60
Potential Pandemic Threats and Preparedness 62
Research Directions and Innovations in Prevention and Control 64
CONCLUSION 66

INTRODUCTION

Avian influenza, frequently referred to as bird flu, is a highly contagious viral virus that mostly affects birds, including domestic poultry and wild birds. While most variants of avian influenza viruses produce only minor sickness in birds, some strains, such as H5N1 and H7N9, can cause serious disease in both birds and humans.

This section provides a full introduction to avian influenza, including its background, previous outbreaks, and the necessity of understanding and controlling this disease in contemporary times.

A Brief Overview of Avian Influenza

Avian influenza is caused by influenza A viruses, which belong to the family Orthomyxoviridae. These viruses are categorized into subgroups based on two surface proteins:

hemagglutinin (HA) and neuraminidase (NA). There are 18 identified HA subtypes and 11 NA subtypes, giving birth to diverse combinations or strains of avian influenza viruses. Among these, several strains have the ability to infect humans and cause serious respiratory disease.

Avian influenza viruses primarily circulate among wild water birds, such as ducks, geese, and shorebirds, which act as natural reservoirs. Domestic fowl, including chickens, turkeys, and ducks, can also be infected by avian influenza viruses, leading to outbreaks in poultry farms.

Transmission of the virus between birds can occur through direct contact with infected birds or their droppings, contaminated feed or water, and contact with contaminated surfaces.

Historical Background and Outbreaks

The history of avian influenza dates back to the early 20th century, when the first recorded outbreak of avian influenza in poultry was reported in Italy in 1878. Since then, multiple outbreaks of avian influenza have been observed globally, affecting both domestic and wild bird populations. One of the most prominent outbreaks happened in 1997, when the H5N1 strain of avian influenza emerged in Hong Kong and infected humans for the first time, raising fears about its pandemic potential.

Subsequent outbreaks of avian influenza, including those caused by other strains such as H7N9 and H5N8, have continued to pose serious dangers to animal and public health. These outbreaks have resulted in extensive economic losses in the poultry business, trade restrictions on poultry products, and, in some cases, human fatalities. The recurring pattern of avian influenza outbreaks highlights the significance of continued surveillance, preventive, and control strategies to limit the burden of the disease.

The Importance of Understanding Avian Influenza Today

Understanding avian influenza is vital for various reasons. Firstly, avian influenza poses a threat to animal health, notably in the poultry industry, where outbreaks can lead to large economic losses due to death, reduced egg production, and trade restrictions. Secondly, avian influenza viruses have the ability to transcend the species barrier and infect people, producing serious respiratory illness and, in some cases, death. Thirdly, avian influenza viruses have the ability to undergo genetic reassortment or mutation, giving rise to new strains with pandemic potential.

In recent years, efforts to study and control avian influenza have escalated, spurred by an understanding of its public health significance and the need to prevent future outbreaks and pandemics. These activities comprise surveillance of avian influenza viruses in both birds and humans, research on the virology and epidemiology of the virus, the development of vaccines and antiviral medications, and the implementation of biosecurity measures in poultry production systems. Additionally, promoting awareness among healthcare experts, poultry workers, and the general public about the risks connected with avian influenza is vital for early detection and response to outbreaks.

In summary, avian influenza is a serious worldwide health concern due to its ability to create devastating epidemics in poultry and represent a threat to human health. Understanding the nature of avian influenza, its historical context, and the need for proactive efforts in surveillance, prevention, and control is vital for limiting the hazards associated with this disease.

CHAPTER 1

UNDERSTANDING AVIAN INFLUENZA VIRUS

Avian influenza virus (AIV) is a type of influenza virus that mostly infects birds, including domestic poultry and wild birds. Understanding the structure, features, strains, subtypes, transmission, and spread of the avian influenza virus is critical for efficient surveillance, prevention, and control of the illness.

Structure and Characteristics of the Avian Influenza Virus

The avian influenza virus belongs to the family Orthomyxoviridae and the genus Influenzavirus A. Like other influenza viruses, AIVs are enclosed, single-stranded RNA viruses with a segmented genome. The genome includes eight segments that encode several viral proteins, including hemagglutinin (HA), neuraminidase (NA), nucleoprotein (NP), matrix protein (M), nonstructural protein (NS), and polymerase proteins (PB1, PB2, and PA). Among these proteins, HA and NA are the primary surface glycoproteins responsible for viral attachment, entrance, and release from host cells.

The HA protein enhances the binding of the virus to sialic acid receptors on host cells, allowing the virus to enter the cell and commence infection. The NA protein, on the other hand, cleaves sialic acid residues from newly produced viral particles, accelerating the discharge of virions from infected cells and preventing their agglomeration. Other viral proteins, such as NP and polymerase proteins, perform critical roles in viral replication, transcription, and assembly.

Avian influenza viruses are categorized into subtypes based on the antigenic characteristics of the HA and NA proteins. To date, 18 HA subtypes (H1–H18) and 11 NA subtypes

(N1–N11) have been found, giving rise to diverse combinations or strains of AIVs. Among these subtypes, the H5 and H7 subtypes are of particular concern due to their ability to cause serious sickness in both birds and people.

Different strains and subtypes

Avian influenza viruses demonstrate a wide variety of genetic variation, with distinct strains and subtypes circulating among bird populations globally. Some variants, such as H5N1 and H7N9, have caused outbreaks in poultry and sporadic cases of human infection, leading to concerns about their pandemic potential. Other strains, like H9N2 and H5N8, have also been involved in outbreaks in poultry but have often produced milder sickness in people.

The classification of AIV strains and subtypes is based on genetic and antigenic investigations of viral isolates collected from birds and humans. Each subtype is named by its mix of HA and NA proteins, such as H5N1 or H7N9. The genetic diversity of AIVs is linked to the high mutation rate of the virus, which allows it to adapt to varied host species and conditions.

Transmission and Spread of Avian Influenza

Avian influenza viruses are usually transmitted among birds by direct contact with infected birds or their secretions, such as saliva, dung, and respiratory droplets. The virus can also spread indirectly through infected surfaces, water sources, feeds, and equipment. Wild birds, particularly waterfowl and shorebirds, are natural reservoirs of AIVs and play a significant role in the global transmission of the virus through migration and movement patterns.

In addition to bird-to-bird transmission, avian influenza viruses can occasionally infect mammals, including people, pigs, and other animals. Human infections with AIVs often occur through intimate contact with infected birds or their habitats, such as poultry farms or live bird markets. While most human infections result in moderate respiratory illness, some AIV strains, such as H5N1 and H7N9, have caused severe respiratory disease with significant fatality rates.

In summary, understanding the structure, features, strains, subtypes, transmission, and spread of the avian influenza virus is critical for efficient surveillance, prevention, and control of the illness.

By monitoring AIVs in bird populations, adopting biosecurity measures in poultry production systems, and raising awareness among healthcare professionals and the public, efforts can be taken to limit the hazards associated with avian influenza and avoid future outbreaks.

CHAPTER 2

SYMPTOMS AND CLINICAL MANIFESTATIONS

Avian influenza, caused by distinct strains of the avian influenza virus (AIV), presents variably in bird species and humans. Understanding the indications, symptoms, and clinical presentations is critical for the early detection, diagnosis, and management of the condition.

Signs and Symptoms in Avian Species

Avian influenza can induce a range of clinical signs and symptoms in infected birds, depending on the virus strain, host species, and environmental conditions. In poultry, frequent indications of avian influenza include the following:

1. Respiratory Symptoms: Infected birds may develop respiratory indications such as coughing, sneezing, nasal discharge, and trouble breathing. Respiratory distress and gasping for air may occur in severe situations.

2. Decreased Egg Production: Egg-laying chickens may have an abrupt decline in egg production or produce eggs with atypical shells, such as soft-shelled or malformed eggs.

3. Swelling and Cyanosis: Some birds may develop swelling of the head, comb, and wattles, as well as cyanosis (bluish staining) of the wattles, comb, and legs due to insufficient oxygenation.

4. Nervous Signs: Neurological signs such as tremors, paralysis, ataxia (lack of coordination), and torticollis (twisted neck) may occur in infected birds, particularly with highly virulent strains of AIV.

5. Sudden Death: In severe situations, avian influenza can cause sudden death without any preceding clinical indications, especially in poultry flocks with high morbidity and mortality rates.

It is vital to highlight that the severity of clinical indications and results can vary greatly among avian species and individual birds within a flock. Factors such as age, immunological status, concomitant infections, and environmental stresses can impact the development of clinical disease.

Human Infections: Symptoms and Complications

While most human infections with avian influenza viruses result in moderate respiratory illness or asymptomatic infection, some strains, such as H5N1 and H7N9, can cause severe disease with high fatality rates. The symptoms of avian influenza in humans are similar to those of seasonal influenza and may include:

1. Fever: Fever is a frequent symptom of avian influenza and is often accompanied by chills, body pains, and weariness.

2. Respiratory Symptoms: Infected patients may have a cough, sore throat, nasal congestion, and difficulty breathing. Severe instances might develop into pneumonia and acute respiratory distress syndrome (ARDS).

Some patients may have gastrointestinal symptoms such as nausea, vomiting, diarrhea, and abdominal discomfort.

3. Systemic Symptoms: In addition to respiratory and gastrointestinal symptoms, avian influenza can induce systemic signs such as headache, muscle discomfort, and malaise.

4. Consequences: Severe instances of avian influenza can lead to consequences such as respiratory failure, multiorgan dysfunction, sepsis, and death. Certain risk factors, including underlying medical disorders (e.g., diabetes, cardiovascular disease) and immunosuppression, may raise the likelihood of severe disease and bad outcomes.

Variations in Clinical Presentation

The clinical manifestation of avian influenza can vary depending on several factors, including the viral strain, host vulnerability, and immunological response. Highly pathogenic avian influenza (HPAI) viruses often produce more severe disease with significant fatality rates in both avian and human populations. In contrast, low-pathogenic avian influenza (LPAI) viruses may induce mild or asymptomatic infections in birds and humans.

Furthermore, avian influenza viruses can undergo genetic reassortment and mutation, leading to the formation of novel strains with altered virulence, transmissibility, and clinical features. Monitoring the genetic and antigenic development of AIVs is critical for understanding the epidemiology of the disease and identifying possible public health hazards.

In summary, avian influenza can appear with a wide spectrum of clinical signs and symptoms in both avian species and humans. Early detection, surveillance, and control techniques are crucial for preventing the spread of the virus and reducing the impact of outbreaks on animal and public health.

CHAPTER 3

DIAGNOSIS AND DETECTION

Avian influenza presents considerable hurdles in diagnosis and detection due to its various strains, varying clinical presentations, and potential for fast dissemination. Accurate and fast diagnosis is critical for adopting effective control measures, avoiding transmission, and reducing the effects of epidemics on animal and public health.

Laboratory Tests for Avian Influenza

Laboratory diagnosis of avian influenza principally relies on the detection and characterization of the influenza virus, notably its hemagglutinin (HA) and neuraminidase (NA) proteins. Several laboratory approaches are performed for avian influenza diagnosis, including:

1. Virus Isolation: Virus isolation requires inoculating clinical materials (e.g., swabs, tissues) onto susceptible cell cultures or embryonated chicken eggs to isolate and propagate the virus. Isolated viruses are then analyzed by serological and molecular methods.

2. Reverse Transcription Polymerase Chain Reaction (RT-PCR): RT-PCR is a sensitive and specific molecular approach used to detect and amplify viral RNA sequences. It enables the quick identification and subtyping of avian influenza viruses based on their genomic markers.

3. Serological Tests: Serological assays, such as enzyme-linked immunosorbent assays (ELISA) and hemagglutination inhibition (HI) assays, detect antibodies produced in response to avian influenza virus infection. Serological tests are important for the surveillance and monitoring of viral circulation in chicken populations.

4. Antigen Detection: Rapid antigen detection procedures, including immunofluorescence assays (IFA) and lateral flow immunoassays (LFIA), identify viral antigens directly from clinical specimens, enabling quick results for on-site diagnosis.

5. Genetic Sequencing: Genetic sequencing enables the whole or partial sequencing of the viral genome, providing crucial information on the virus's origin, genetic variety, and possible pathogenicity.

Diagnostic Methods in Humans and Animals

In humans, the diagnosis of avian influenza relies on clinical evaluation, laboratory testing, and epidemiological study. Clinical specimens, such as respiratory secretions, throat swabs, and blood samples, are taken from suspected cases for virological and serological testing. RT-PCR and viral culture are routinely used laboratory procedures for diagnosing human instances of avian influenza.

In animals, particularly poultry and wild birds, surveillance and monitoring programs are vital for the early detection of avian influenza outbreaks. Veterinarians and animal health specialists employ a mix of clinical examination, laboratory testing, and risk assessment to diagnose avian influenza in birds. Post-mortem exams, serological testing, and molecular diagnostics are key components of avian influenza surveillance in avian populations.

Challenges in Early Detection and Diagnosis

Despite breakthroughs in diagnostic tools, several hurdles continue in the early identification and diagnosis of avian influenza:

1. Cross-reactivity: Avian influenza viruses may cross-react with other respiratory infections, resulting in false-positive or false-negative results in diagnostic testing.

2. Antigenic Drift and Shift: The genetic heterogeneity of avian influenza viruses, resulting from antigenic drift and shift, creates difficulty in creating diagnostic assays that can accurately detect newly emerging strains.

3. Sampling Issues: Inadequate sample collection, storage, and transport can limit the sensitivity and reliability of diagnostic tests, leading to erroneous results.

4. Limited Access to Laboratory Facilities: Resource constraints, particularly in low-resource settings, may limit access to laboratory facilities able to perform advanced diagnostic tests for avian influenza.

5. Monitoring Gaps: Gaps in monitoring systems and underreporting of avian influenza illnesses in both animals and people limit the early diagnosis and containment of outbreaks.

Despite these limitations, continued research efforts and coordination between public health agencies, veterinary authorities, and research institutions are crucial for strengthening diagnostic skills and enhancing worldwide preparedness for avian influenza epidemics.

Early diagnosis and prompt reaction are essential components of effective disease control methods aimed at reducing the effects of avian influenza on global health security.

CHAPTER 4

PREVENTION AND CONTROL MEASURES

Avian influenza, with its potential to produce severe outbreaks in poultry and sporadic human infections, demands comprehensive prevention and control strategies at both the animal and human levels.

Effective solutions comprise immunization, biosecurity techniques, and public health activities targeted at reducing transmission and decreasing the burden of the disease.

Vaccination Strategies for Poultry

1. Inactivated Vaccines: Inactivated avian influenza vaccines are routinely used in poultry to establish protective immunity against circulating viral strains. These vaccinations include dead viral particles and are administered via injection or spray. Inactivated vaccines are helpful in lowering clinical symptoms and mortality rates in vaccinated birds.

2. Live Attenuated Vaccines: Live attenuated vaccines, developed from weakened strains of the avian influenza virus, generate powerful immune responses in vaccinated chickens. These vaccinations are delivered orally or via nasal drops and confer both humoral and cellular immunity against avian influenza. Live-attenuated vaccinations are particularly useful for preventing highly pathogenic avian influenza (HPAI) outbreaks in poultry.

3. Vector Vaccines: Vector vaccines utilize harmless viral vectors, such as the fowlpox virus or Newcastle disease virus, to deliver avian influenza antigens to vaccinated birds. Vector vaccines are useful in inducing protective immune responses and can be delivered via spray or in ovo immunization procedures.

4. Strain-individual vaccines: Avian influenza vaccines are tailored to individual virus strains based on antigenic characterization and genetic study. Vaccination regimens may use monovalent or multivalent vaccines targeting prevalent avian influenza subtypes to give the best protection to poultry populations.

5. Compliance with Vaccination Schedules: Adherence to approved vaccination schedules is vital for guaranteeing the success of avian influenza immunization programs. Poultry farmers must maintain accurate records of vaccine administration and evaluate vaccine efficacy using serological testing and surveillance.

Biosecurity Measures in Poultry Farms

1. Farm Hygiene and Sanitation: Proper sanitation procedures, including cleaning and disinfection of chicken houses, equipment, and vehicles, help limit the risk of avian influenza transmission inside and between farms.

2. Restricted Access: Implementing tight biosecurity policies, such as restricting access to poultry farms, minimizing visitor traffic, and establishing designated entry points, minimizes the likelihood of spreading the avian influenza virus to sensitive bird populations.

3. Separation of Poultry Flocks: Segregating poultry flocks based on age, health state, and species decreases the spread of avian influenza within production facilities. Physical barriers, such as fences and biosecurity zones, help limit contact between various bird populations.

4. Control of Wild Bird Access: Limiting contact between domestic poultry and wild birds, which can serve as reservoirs for the avian influenza virus, minimizes the risk of introduction and transmission of the virus to poultry farms. Measures may include netting, bird-proofing structures, and habitat management.

5. Surveillance and Monitoring: Regular surveillance for avian influenza by active monitoring of chicken health, mortality, and clinical symptoms permits early discovery of outbreaks and facilitates rapid implementation of control measures.

Public Health Measures for Preventing Human Transmission

1. Surveillance and Early Detection: Public health agencies conduct surveillance for human instances of avian influenza. Timely diagnosis and reporting facilitate the implementation of infection control measures and public health interventions.

2. Personal Protective Equipment (PPE): Healthcare personnel and individuals at risk of exposure to the avian influenza virus, such as poultry workers and travelers to impacted areas, should use proper PPE, including gloves, masks, and protective clothes, to limit the risk of infection.

3. Infection Control Measures: Implementation of infection control measures, such as hand hygiene, respiratory etiquette, and environmental sanitation, lowers the danger of human-to-human transmission of the avian influenza virus.

4. Health Education and Risk Communication: Public health authorities distribute correct information regarding avian influenza risks, preventative tactics, and epidemic response measures to the public, healthcare providers, and stakeholders. Clear communication increases community engagement and compliance with prescribed measures.

5. Antiviral Treatment and Vaccination: Antiviral drugs, such as neuraminidase inhibitors (e.g., oseltamivir, zanamivir), may be given for the treatment of human avian influenza infections. Vaccination against seasonal influenza decreases the likelihood of co-infection with avian influenza virus strains and mitigates the load on healthcare systems during outbreaks.

Comprehensive prevention and control strategies for avian influenza require a multi-sectoral approach requiring coordination between veterinary and public health agencies, poultry producers, healthcare providers, and the community.

Timely implementation of vaccination programs, biosecurity measures, and public health interventions is critical for defending both animal and human health against the threat of avian influenza outbreaks.

CHAPTER 5

TREATMENT AND MANAGEMENT

Avian influenza, particularly the highly pathogenic forms, presents considerable problems in terms of treatment and management due to its rapid progression, potential for severe consequences, and limited efficacy of antiviral drugs.

Effective management options attempt to alleviate symptoms, prevent complications, and control the transmission of the virus in both avian and human populations.

Antiviral Medications for Avian Influenza

Antiviral drugs have a significant role in the treatment of avian influenza, especially in severe cases or those at high risk of sequelae. The principal antiviral medications used in the management of avian influenza include:

1. Neuraminidase Inhibitors: Oseltamivir (Tamiflu) and zanamivir (Relenza) are neuraminidase inhibitors that interfere with the release of offspring viruses from infected cells, therefore limiting viral replication and dissemination. These drugs are most effective when begun early in the course of sickness and have been found to lessen the severity and duration of symptoms.

2. Adamantanes: Amantadine and rimantadine are adamantane derivatives that inhibit the viral M2 ion channel protein, hence preventing viral replication. However, the widespread appearance of adamantane-resistant strains has reduced their utility in the treatment of avian influenza and other influenza viruses.

3. Peramivir: Peramivir is an intravenous neuraminidase inhibitor licensed for the treatment of influenza, particularly avian influenza, in some countries. It offers an alternative treatment option for those unable to tolerate oral drugs or those with severe illnesses necessitating hospitalization.

4. Baloxavir Marboxil: Baloxavir marboxil is a novel antiviral drug that inhibits the cap-dependent endonuclease activity of the viral polymerase, hence preventing viral replication. It is approved for the treatment of influenza in several countries and may offer benefits in the management of avian influenza, particularly in cases of oseltamivir-resistant viruses.

Supportive care for infected individuals

In addition to antiviral medication, supportive care measures are crucial for controlling avian influenza infections and minimizing consequences. Supportive care interventions may include:

1. Fluid and Electrolyte Management: Maintaining proper hydration and electrolyte balance is critical, especially in cases of severe dehydration owing to fever, vomiting, or diarrhea.

2. Respiratory Support: Patients with severe respiratory symptoms may require supplementary oxygen therapy, mechanical ventilation, or extracorporeal membrane oxygenation (ECMO) in critical care settings.

3. Fever Management: Antipyretic drugs such as acetaminophen or ibuprofen might help relieve fever and discomfort in infected patients.

4. Nutritional Support: Adequate nutrition is vital for boosting immune function and facilitating healing. Nutritional supplements or enteral feeding may be necessary for those unable to tolerate oral consumption.

Strategies for Managing Outbreaks in Poultry and Humans

Controlling epidemics of avian influenza involves a multi-faceted approach involving veterinary and public health agencies, poultry producers, healthcare professionals, and the community. Key measures for handling epidemics include the following:

1. Surveillance and Early Detection: Robust surveillance systems are necessary for the early detection of avian influenza epidemics in poultry populations. Timely reporting of suspected cases to veterinary authorities permits prompt response and control measures.

2. Quarantine and Movement Restrictions: Implementing quarantine measures and movement restrictions for afflicted poultry farms or regions can help limit the transmission of the virus to unaffected areas. Culling diseased and at-risk birds may be necessary to prevent further transmission.

3. Biosecurity Measures: Strict biosecurity standards, including better cleaning and disinfection methods, restricted access to poultry facilities, and correct disposal of infected materials, are crucial for preventing the introduction and spread of avian influenza on farms.

4. Mass Vaccination Programs: The vaccination of chicken populations, particularly in countries with endemic avian influenza, can help lower the prevalence and severity of outbreaks. Vaccination tactics target specific strains of the avian influenza virus circulating in chicken populations.

5. Public Health Interventions: Public health measures, such as surveillance of human cases, contact tracing, isolation of infected individuals, and promotion of personal hygiene and respiratory etiquette, are essential for preventing human-to-human transmission of avian influenza viruses, particularly those with pandemic potential.

In conclusion, successful management of avian influenza requires a comprehensive approach involving antiviral medicine, supportive care, and public health activities.

Timely deployment of control measures, together with continued surveillance and research activities, is critical for limiting the impact of avian influenza on both animal and human health.

CHAPTER 6

GLOBAL SURVEILLANCE AND RESPONSE

Bird influenza is a significant public health problem with the potential for broad transmission and devastating effects on both bird and human populations. As such, robust global surveillance and response procedures are necessary for early identification, fast containment, and effective control of avian influenza outbreaks.

This chapter analyzes the international efforts in monitoring avian influenza, coordinated response systems, and the challenges and potential in global surveillance.

International Efforts in Monitoring Avian Influenza

1. World Health Organization (WHO): The WHO plays a vital role in global efforts to monitor and respond to avian influenza. Through the Global Influenza Programme, the WHO coordinates surveillance activities, offers technical guidance, and enables the sharing of information and resources among member states.

2. World Organisation for Animal Health (OIE): The OIE is responsible for coordinating international efforts to control animal illnesses, particularly avian influenza. The OIE's World Animal Health Information System (WAHIS) provides a framework for reporting and monitoring outbreaks of avian influenza in animal populations worldwide.

3. Food and Agriculture Organization (FAO): The FAO partners with the WHO and OIE to address the human and animal health aspects of avian influenza. The FAO's Emergency Prevention System for Transboundary Animal and Plant Pests and Diseases (EMPRES) provides support for surveillance, early warning, and response efforts in impacted regions.

4. Global Influenza Surveillance and Response System (GISRS): GISRS is a network of laboratories and monitoring stations coordinated by the WHO. It monitors the transmission of influenza viruses, especially avian influenza, allows the interchange of influenza data and specimens, and gives advice on vaccine strain selection.

Collaborative Response Mechanisms

1. Pandemic Preparedness and Reaction: Recognizing the potential for avian influenza viruses to produce pandemics in humans, countries have developed pandemic preparedness plans that detail tactics for surveillance, containment, and reaction. These strategies emphasize coordination across public health, veterinary, and other relevant sectors at national and international levels.

2. Worldwide Health Regulations (IHR): The IHR, established by the WHO, provides a legislative framework for the prevention and control of public health emergencies of worldwide relevance, including avian influenza outbreaks. Member governments are expected to notifythe WHO of certain incidents, including outbreaks of avian influenza, and to collaborate in response activities.

3. Global Outbreak Alert and Response Network (GOARN): GOARN is a network of institutions and professionals dedicated to facilitating the quick detection and response to outbreaks of infectious illnesses, particularly avian influenza. It offers technical support, dispatches reaction teams, and coordinates international aid during public health emergencies.

Challenges and Opportunities in Global Surveillance

1. Limited Surveillance Capacity: Many nations, particularly in low-resource contexts, confront difficulty in developing and maintaining adequate surveillance systems for avian influenza. Limited laboratory capacity, weak reporting infrastructure, and competing goals contribute to gaps in surveillance data.

2. Cross-Species Transmission: Avian influenza viruses have the ability to infect several species, including birds, animals, and humans. Monitoring and detecting cross-species transmission events require coordinated monitoring efforts across the human and animal health sectors, as well as greater collaboration between national and international authorities.

3. Antigenic Drift and Shift: Avian influenza viruses undergo regular genetic alterations through antigenic drift and shift, which can affect their virulence, transmissibility, and ability to evade immune responses. Surveillance systems must continuously monitor circulating strains and assess their pandemic potential.

4. Global Health Security: Avian influenza represents a substantial danger to global health security due to its pandemic potential and potential for devastating economic and social ramifications. Strengthening global surveillance and response capacity is vital for reducing the effects of avian influenza outbreaks and averting future pandemics.

In conclusion, global surveillance and response efforts are crucial for detecting, monitoring, and controlling avian influenza epidemics.

Collaboration between international organizations, national governments, research institutions, and other stakeholders is crucial for effectively addressing the problems posed by avian influenza and maintaining public health on a worldwide scale.

CHAPTER 7

PUBLIC HEALTH PREPAREDNESS

Public health preparation is vital for effectively reacting to the threat of avian influenza epidemics and reducing their impact on human populations.

National and regional governments, along with healthcare providers and community organizations, play essential roles in formulating and implementing preparation plans, increasing monitoring capacities, and educating the public about avian influenza risks and preventative techniques.

National and Regional Preparedness Plans

National governments, in partnership with international health agencies such as the World Health Organization

(WHO) and the Food and Agriculture Organization (FAO), construct comprehensive preparedness plans to manage avian influenza epidemics. These plans often include:

1. Surveillance Systems: Establishing and maintaining robust surveillance systems to detect avian influenza epidemics in both poultry and humans. Surveillance data informs response efforts and promotes prompt action.

2. Response Protocols: Developing response protocols for managing avian influenza epidemics, including measures for quick containment, risk communication, and resource mobilization. Clear lines of communication and coordination among government agencies, healthcare providers, and other stakeholders are vital.

2. Stockpiling of Medical Supplies: Stockpiling antiviral drugs, personal protective equipment (PPE), and other medical supplies to ensure speedy access during outbreaks. Maintaining appropriate supplies of vaccinations and antiviral medications is critical for protecting healthcare professionals and high-risk populations.

3. Vaccination Campaigns: Implementing vaccination campaigns for at-risk populations, such as poultry workers, healthcare personnel, and individuals in high-transmission areas. Vaccination strategies attempt to prevent human illnesses and restrict the spread of avian influenza viruses.

4. Capacity Building: Strengthening laboratory capacities, healthcare infrastructure, and emergency response skills to effectively handle avian influenza outbreaks. Training programs for healthcare personnel and emergency responders boost preparedness and response efforts.

Role of Healthcare Providers in Surveillance and Response

Healthcare practitioners have a crucial role in influenza surveillance, diagnosis, and treatment, as well as in educating the public about prevention measures. Key roles include:

1. Surveillance and Reporting: Healthcare providers are responsible for recognizing and reporting suspected cases of avian influenza in humans. Timely reporting to public health authorities improves early detection and response activities.

2. Clinical Management: Healthcare personnel are taught to recognize the signs and symptoms of avian influenza in patients presenting with respiratory disease. Prompt diagnosis and appropriate therapy in suspected cases are critical for limiting disease severity and preventing consequences.

3. Infection control procedures: hospital facilities adopt severe infection control procedures to limit the spread of avian influenza within hospital settings. These procedures include the isolation of suspected cases, the use of PPE, and adherence to hand hygiene protocols.

4. Risk Communication: Healthcare providers communicate with patients, families, and communities about avian influenza dangers, preventive measures, and treatment options. Clear and accurate information helps ease anxieties and promotes adherence to prescribed actions.

Community Education and Awareness Programs

Community education and awareness activities are key components of public health preparedness measures for avian influenza. These programs aim to:

1. Raise Awareness: Educate the public on the hazards of avian influenza, modes of transmission, and preventive measures, including proper hygiene practices and avoidance of contact with sick or dead birds.

2. Promote Preparedness: Encourage people and families to build preparedness plans for avian influenza epidemics, including stockpiling vital supplies, forming emergency communication plans, and remaining updated about local health advisories.

3. Address Misconceptions: Counter misinformation and dispel myths about avian influenza through focused educational initiatives. Providing accurate information helps establish trust and confidence in public health authorities and improves adherence to prescribed actions.

4. Foster Community Resilience: Engage communities in joint efforts to prevent and respond to avian influenza epidemics. Community-based groups, religious institutions, and local leaders play crucial roles in distributing information, assisting vulnerable populations, and creating solidarity during times of crisis.

In conclusion, public health preparation is vital for efficiently reacting to avian influenza epidemics and maintaining population health. National and regional governments, healthcare providers, and community organizations must work together to establish and implement preparation plans, increase surveillance capacities, and educate the public about avian influenza dangers and preventative techniques.

By developing resilient health systems and increasing community engagement, we can limit the impact of avian influenza and protect the well-being of individuals and communities globally.

CHAPTER 8

ONE HEALTH APPROACH

The One Health approach is a holistic paradigm that recognizes the connection between human health, animal health, and environmental health. It emphasizes the significance of teamwork and interdisciplinary efforts to overcome complex health concerns, such as zoonotic illnesses, antibiotic resistance, and environmental pollution.

This section covers the fundamentals of the One Health approach, its significance in defending public health, and offers case studies and success stories that indicate its effectiveness in addressing global health problems.

Integrating human, animal, and environmental health

The One Health concept recognizes that the health of humans, animals, and ecosystems is inextricably interrelated and interdependent. Key components of the One Health framework include:

1. Zoonotic Disease Surveillance: Monitoring and surveillance of zoonotic illnesses, which begin in animals but can transfer to people, are critical for early diagnosis and response. Examples of zoonotic diseases include avian influenza, Ebola virus disease, and COVID-19.

2. Antimicrobial Resistance (AMR): Addressing antimicrobial resistance requires a One Health strategy that recognizes the interconnection of human and animal antibiotic usage as well as environmental factors contributing to the spread of resistant microorganisms. Collaborative efforts are needed to promote appropriate antimicrobial use in healthcare, agriculture, and veterinary contexts.

3. Environmental Health: Protecting environmental health is vital for preventing the emergence and spread of infectious diseases and reducing the impact of environmental toxins on human and animal populations. Addressing concerns such as air and water pollution, deforestation, and climate change requires interdisciplinary methods that address the health of ecosystems and biodiversity.

Importance of Collaboration and Interdisciplinary Efforts

The success of the One Health strategy relies on collaboration among many stakeholders, including:

1. Healthcare Professionals: Physicians, veterinarians, epidemiologists, and other healthcare professionals collaborate to solve health concerns that cross human and animal populations. Interdisciplinary training programs and cooperative research efforts foster cross-sectoral collaboration and knowledge sharing.

1. Public Health Agencies: National and international public health agencies play essential roles in coordinating One Health efforts, facilitating data sharing, and providing technical expertise and resources. Collaboration between public health agencies, animal health authorities, and environmental agencies increases surveillance and response capacities.

2. Academic Institutions: Universities and research institutions contribute to One Health research and education, enabling multidisciplinary collaboration among students, faculty, and researchers. One Health programs and initiatives prepare the next generation of professionals to handle complex health concerns through integrated methods.

3. Government Agencies: Governments provide rules and regulations to promote One Health programs, allocate financing for research and surveillance activities, and facilitate cross-sectoral collaboration. Interministerial task forces and advisory committees foster collaboration between health, agriculture, the environment, and other related sectors.

Case Studies and Success Stories

This section highlights case studies and success stories that indicate the effectiveness of the One Health approach in tackling real-world health challenges:

1. Control of Zoonotic Diseases: Case studies indicate how integrated surveillance and control techniques have successfully prevented and contained zoonotic disease outbreaks, such as the eradication of rabies in specific regions and the control of Ebola epidemics through coordinated response efforts.

2. AMR Mitigation: Success stories illustrate attempts to address antimicrobial resistance through collaborative approaches that promote responsible antimicrobial use in human and animal healthcare settings, limit antibiotic misuse in agriculture, and raise knowledge about the problem of AMR.

3. Environmental Health Interventions: Examples of environmental health interventions show the influence of pollution control measures, habitat restoration projects, and sustainable land use practices on improving public health outcomes and conserving ecosystem integrity.

In conclusion, the One Health approach offers a comprehensive framework for solving complex health concerns by combining human, animal, and environmental health factors. Collaboration and interdisciplinary efforts are vital for successful disease surveillance, prevention, and control, as well as for improving environmental sustainability and resilience.

By adopting the ideas of One Health and promoting multisectoral relationships, we can achieve a healthier and more sustainable future for everybody

CHAPTER 9

FUTURE PERSPECTIVES AND EMERGING CHALLENGES

As our understanding of avian influenza continues to evolve, it is crucial to anticipate future trends, problems, and possibilities in the field. This section covers the evolutionary tendencies in avian influenza viruses, potential pandemic dangers, preparatory measures, and upcoming research areas and developments in prevention and control tactics.

Evolutionary Trends in the Avian Influenza Virus

Avian influenza viruses demonstrate a remarkable ability to develop and adapt, offering persistent problems for disease surveillance, prevention, and control. Key evolutionary trends include:

1. Genetic Drift and Shift: Avian influenza viruses undergo regular genetic changes and reassortments, leading to the formation of novel strains with altered antigenic characteristics. Genetic drift resulted in modest changes in viral surface proteins, while genetic drift can lead to the formation of highly virulent viruses with pandemic potential.

2. Host Range Expansion: Avian influenza viruses have the capacity to infect a wide range of avian and mammalian species, including domestic poultry, wild birds, and occasionally humans. Zoonotic transmission events, where viruses adapt to infect and disseminate among people, pose enormous public health hazards and can potentially lead to worldwide pandemics.

3. Ecological Factors: Environmental factors, such as climate change, habitat destruction, and wildlife commerce, influence the spread and transmission dynamics of avian influenza viruses. Changes in migratory patterns, habitat loss, and human encroachment into wildlife areas might facilitate interspecies transmission and overflow events.

Potential Pandemic Threats and Preparedness

The continued threat of avian influenza pandemics needs continuous awareness and preparatory activities to limit the consequences of prospective outbreaks. Key considerations include:

1. Emerging Strains: Monitoring avian influenza viruses for genetic alterations and enhanced pathogenicity is critical for the early detection of emerging strains with pandemic potential. Surveillance efforts should focus on high-risk regions and species, including poultry farms, live bird markets, and wild bird populations.

2. Pandemic Preparedness Plans: National and international pandemic preparedness plans detail measures for quick reaction and containment in the event of an avian influenza pandemic. Preparedness strategies include stockpiling antiviral drugs, developing candidate vaccines, strengthening laboratory capacity for diagnostic testing, and implementing public health interventions like social distancing measures and travel restrictions.

3. Global Cooperation: International collaboration and information sharing are important for effective pandemic preparedness and response. Platforms such as the World Health Organization (WHO), the Food and Agriculture Organization (FAO), and the World Organisation for Animal Health (OIE) facilitate coordination among countries, promote data sharing, and support capacity-building initiatives in regions at high risk of avian influenza outbreaks.

Research Directions and Innovations in Prevention and Control

Advancements in science and technology play a critical role in expanding our understanding of avian influenza and generating creative ways for prevention and control. Key research directions and innovations include the following:

1. Vaccine Development: Ongoing research efforts focus on the development of next-generation vaccines that give broader protection against varied strains of avian influenza viruses. Novel vaccination platforms, such as vectored vaccines, virus-like particles (VLPs), and recombinant protein vaccines, hold potential for enhancing vaccine efficacy and cross-protection.

2. Antiviral Therapeutics: The discovery and development of new antiviral medications targeting distinct stages of the viral replication cycle are vital for treating avian influenza infections and lowering disease severity. Research activities aim to identify novel antiviral agents with broad-spectrum efficacy against different influenza virus strains, including highly dangerous avian influenza viruses.

3. Surveillance Technologies: Advances in molecular diagnostics, next-generation sequencing (NGS), and analytics enable rapid and precise detection, characterization, and surveillance of avian influenza viruses in both human and animal populations. Real-time genomic surveillance gives crucial insights into viral evolution, transmission dynamics, and the generation of antiviral resistance variants.

In conclusion, the future of avian influenza prevention and control demands a multidimensional approach that blends scientific research, public health preparedness, and worldwide cooperation. By monitoring evolutionary trends, developing pandemic preparedness strategies, and investing in research and innovation, we can effectively limit the hazards presented by avian influenza and defend global health security.

CONCLUSION

As we complete our investigation of avian influenza and its consequences for global health, it is vital to reflect on the key topics presented throughout this thorough book.

This final section presents a recapitulation of essential themes, underlines the significance of vigilance and proactive measures in avian influenza control, and makes a call to action for continuous efforts to improve health and safety in the face of this ongoing threat.

RECAPITULATION OF KEY POINTS

Throughout this book, we have dug into different elements of avian influenza, including its virology, transmission dynamics, clinical manifestations, diagnosis, prevention, treatment, surveillance, and global reaction mechanisms.

KEY POINTS MENTIONED INCLUDE:

Avian influenza viruses belong to the Orthomyxoviridae family and mostly harm birds, with infrequent spillover events resulting in human infections.

Avian influenza viruses are divided into several subtypes based on their surface glycoproteins, hemagglutinin (HA), and neuraminidase (NA), with H5N1 and H7N9 being of particular concern due to their high pathogenicity in birds and potential to cause serious sickness in people.

Avian influenza can show a wide spectrum of symptoms in both avian and human hosts, ranging from mild respiratory disease to severe pneumonia and multi-organ failure.

Early detection and diagnosis of avian influenza infections relies on laboratory testing, including viral isolation, nucleic acid amplification tests (e.g., RT-PCR), serological assays, and genomic sequencing.

Prevention and control techniques involve a One Health approach, incorporating human, animal, and environmental health perspectives. Strategies include immunization, biosecurity measures, public health interventions, antiviral therapy, and global surveillance activities.

International collaboration and coordinated response systems are necessary for efficient pandemic preparedness and response, involving institutions like the WHO, FAO, OIE, and national public health agencies.

IMPORTANCE OF VIGILANCE AND PROACTIVE MEASURES

Avian influenza remains a huge danger to global health security, with the potential to create disastrous outbreaks in poultry and humans alike. The continual evolution and spread of avian influenza viruses underline the significance of monitoring and employing proactive steps to limit the hazards associated with these diseases. By keeping watchful and proactive, we may better predict and respond to new risks, shielding both animal and human populations from the detrimental repercussions of avian influenza outbreaks.

CALL TO ACTION FOR CONTINUED EFFORTS IN AVIAN INFLUENZA CONTROL

As we look to the future, it is evident that the fight against avian influenza requires ongoing commitment and concerted action from all stakeholders involved. Governments, public health agencies, veterinary authorities, healthcare providers, researchers, industry partners, and communities must work together to strengthen surveillance systems, enhance preparedness and response capabilities, and advance research and innovation in avian influenza prevention and control.

A CALL TO ACTION IS ISSUED FOR:

Continued investment in research and development of vaccines, antiviral medicines, diagnostic tools, and surveillance technologies will increase our ability to prevent, detect, and respond to avian influenza epidemics.

Enhanced collaboration and information sharing among countries, regions, and international organizations to support timely and coordinated responses to emerging threats and global health crises.

Greater public awareness and education campaigns to promote understanding of avian influenza threats, preventive measures, and the necessity of One Health approaches in safeguarding human and animal health.

Sustainable agricultural techniques and responsible poultry production systems that prioritize biosecurity, animal welfare, and environmental stewardship will limit the risk of avian influenza transmission and spread.

In conclusion, by being attentive, proactive, and collaborative, we may effectively limit the hazards posed by avian influenza and promote health and safety for all. Together, we can work towards a future where the threat of avian influenza is minimized and the well-being of both humans and animals is preserved.

www.ingramcontent.com/pod-product-compliance
Lightning Source LLC
Chambersburg PA
CBHW051535240526
45471CB00020B/2678